A Complete Guide to Losing Weight with Healthy and Tasty Recipes and a List of Foods that will Help You Activate Sirtuins

10 MINUTES MEALS AMERICA

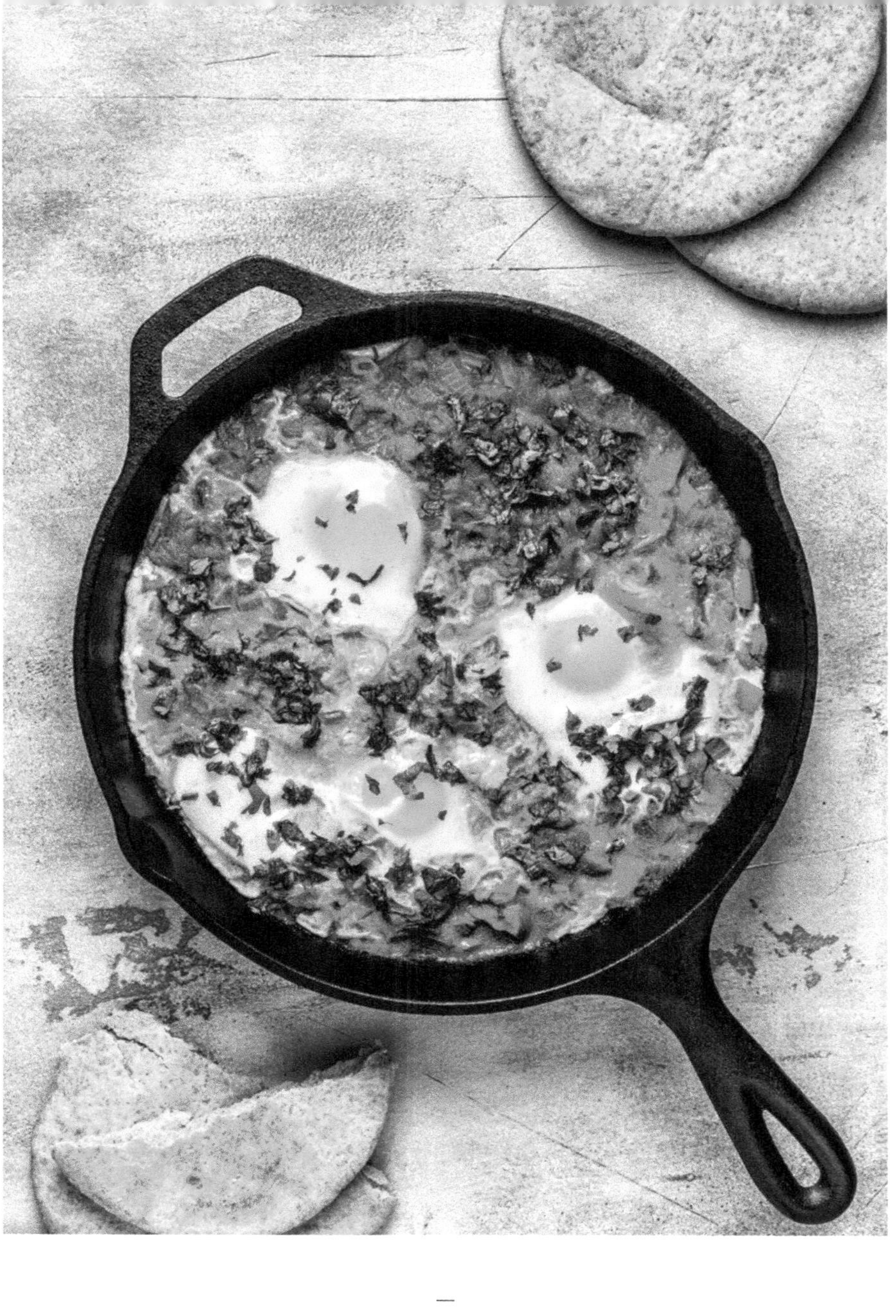

—
2

providing information that is as accurate and reliable as possible. Regardless, purchasing this Book can be seen as consent to the fact that both the publisher and the author of this book are in no way experts on the topics discussed within and that any recommendations or suggestions that are made herein are for entertainment purposes only. Professionals should be consulted as needed prior to undertaking any of the action endorsed herein.

inattention, use, or misuse of the information in question by the reader will render any resulting actions solely under their purview. There are no scenarios in which the publisher or the original author of this work can be in any fashion deemed liable for any hardship or damages that may befall them after undertaking information described herein.

Additionally, the information in the following pages is intended only for informational purposes and should thus be thought of as universal. As befitting its nature, it is presented without assurance regarding its prolonged validity or interim quality. Trademarks that are mentioned are done without written consent and can in no way be considered an endorsement from the trademark holder.

"The Sirtfood Diet is the Newest and Latest Strategy for Health, Nutrition and Weight Loss."

The Sirtfood Diet is the new way to shift weight quickly without radical dieting by activating the same 'skinny gene' pathways usually just induced by exercise and fasting. Certain foods contain chemicals called polyphenols that put mild stress on our cells, turning on genes that mimic the effects of fasting and exercise. Foods rich in polyphenols-including kale, dark chocolate and red wine-trigger the sirtuin pathways that impact metabolism, aging and mood. A diet rich in these sirtfoods kick-starts weight loss without sacrificing muscle, while maintaining optimal health.

supercharge weight loss and help stave off disease with this easy-to-follow diet developed by the experts in nutritional medicine who proved the impact of sirtfoods. Dark chocolate, coffee, kale – these are all foods that activate sirtuins and switch on the so-called 'skinny gene' pathways in the body. The Sirtfood Diet gives you a simple, healthy way of eating for weight loss, delicious easy-to-make recipes and a maintenance plan for prolonged success. The Sirtfood Diet is a diet of inclusion not exclusion, and sirtfoods are widely available and affordable. This is a diet that encourages you to pick up your knife and fork, and enjoy eating delicious healthy food while seeing the health and weight-loss benefits.

HOW IT WORKS

The diet has two easy-to-follow phases:

PHASE 1 This lasts for seven days. During the first three days, you should have three sirtfood green juices and one full meal rich in sirtfoods – a total of 1,000 calories. On days four to seven, you should increase your calorie intake to 1,500 by having two green juices and two meals daily.

balanced sirtfood-rich meals every day, plus one green juice. The two phases can be repeated whenever you like for a fat-loss boost. What happens after the second phase? And is this kind of diet really sustainable? The idea of "sirtifying" meals is for those who have completed phase one and two but still want to continue on the Sirtfood path. It involves taking your favourite dish and giving it a Sirtfood twist. Recipes include everyday favourites such as chicken curry, chilli-con-carne, pizza and pancakes. The Sirtfood Diet is not designed to be a one-off 'diet' but rather a way of life. You are encouraged, once you've completed the first 3 weeks, to continue eating a diet rich in Sirtfoods and to continue drinking your daily green juice. There are now many Sirtfood Diet recipe books available, with recipes for lots more Sirtfood-rich main meals, as well as recipes for alternatives to the green juice and more hints and tips for following the Sirtfood Diet. There are even some recipes for Sirtfood desserts! Phases 1 and 2 can be repeated as and when necessary for a health boost, or if things have gone a bit off track.

GETTING STARTED

Daily juices are essential to the Sirtfood Diet. So, make sure you have a juicer. You'll also need three key ingredients. Matcha is a powdered green tea and an important ingredient in the green juices. It's readily available online, if your local health food shop doesn't stock it. Similarly, lovage – a herb in the green juice recipe – can sometimes seem hard to find. But it's easy to buy seeds online to grow it in a pot on a windowsill. Finally, buckwheat. It's a fantastic alternative to more common grains, but most supermarkets mix buckwheat and wheat in their products. You're more likely to find 100 per cent buckwheat products in your local health food store.

- ✦ Chili pepper
- ✦ Buckwheat
- ✦ Capers
- ✦ Celery
- ✦ Cocoa
- ✦ Coffee
- ✦ Extra virgin olive oil
- ✦ Green tea
- ✦ kale
- ✦ lovage
- ✦ medjool dates
- ✦ parsley
- ✦ red chicory red onion
- ✦ red wine
- ✦ rocket
- ✦ soy
- ✦ strawberries
- ✦ turmeric
- ✦ walnuts

Although these are the top 20 sirtfoods, there are other foods approved for this diet like asparagus, green beans, raspberries, and popcorn. You should probably hit the grocery stores and order yourself a juicer before you give this diet a go. There are quite a few moving parts to the phases and a lot of organization required, but it's meant to be fast acting and last about 21 days.

Week 1:

O Limit your intake to 1000 calories a day ➤ Drink three sirtfood green juices a day ➤ Eat one sirtfood rich meal a day.

Week 2:

O Up your intake to 1500 calories a day
O Drink two sirtfood green juices a day
O Eat two sirtfood-rich meals a day

In the long-term there is no set plan. It's all about adjusting your lifestyle to include as many sirtfoods as possible, which should make you feel healthier and more energetic.

building muscle and suppressing appetite. These include improving memory, helping the body better control blood sugar levels and cleaning up the damage from free radical molecules that can accumulate in cells and lead to cancer and other diseases.

'Substantial observational evidence exists for the beneficial effects of the intake of food and drinks rich in sirtuin activators in decreasing risks of chronic disease,' said Professor Frank Hu, an expert in nutrition and epidemiology at Harvard University in a recent article in the journal Advances in Nutrition. A sirtfood diet is particularly suitable as an anti-aging regime. Although sirtuin activators are found all through the plant kingdom, only certain fruits and vegetables have large enough amounts to count as sirtfoods. Examples include green tea, cocoa powder, the Indian spice turmeric, kale, onions and parsley. Many of the fruit and vegetables on display in supermarkets, such as tomatoes, avocados, bananas, lettuce, kiwis, carrots and cucumber, are actually rather low in sirtuin activators. This doesn't mean that they aren't worth eating, though, as they provide lots of other benefits. The beauty of eating a diet packed sirtfoods on top. Or you could have them in a concentrated way. Adding sirtfoods to say, the 5:2 diet could allow more calories on the low-calorie days. A remarkable finding of one sirtfood diet trial is that participants lost substantial weight without losing muscle. In fact, it was common for participants to actually gain muscle, leading to a more defined and toned look. That's the beauty of sirtfoods; they activate fat burning but also promote muscle growth, maintenance and repair. This is in complete contrast to other diets where weight loss typically comes from both fat and muscle, with the loss of muscle slowing down metabolism and making weight regain more likely

IS THE SIRTFOOD DIET GOOD FOR YOU?

One positive of the diet is that all of the foods you can eat on the plan are good for you, meaning your overall vitamin, mineral and nutrient intake will likely be high. any diet that cuts out entire food groups could be dangerous. 'The idea of switching on your 'skinny gene' is not really backed up by very strong research. The Sirtfood diet overall is pretty restrictive in terms of both foods and calories, which may make it difficult to stick too. There is also no evidence to suggest it's a more effective way to lose weight than any other calorie-controlled diet'. In other words, if you're trying to lose weight, why not eat foods you actually enjoy eating, whilst being mindful of your overall calorie intake?

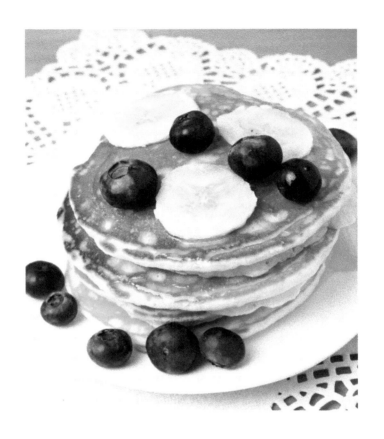

INGREDIENTS:

- 75 g Natural yoghurt o Juice of 1/4 of a lemon o 1 tsp Coriander, chopped o 1 tsp Ground turmeric o 1/2 tsp Mild curry powder
- 100 g Cooked chicken breast, cut into bite-sized pieces o 6 Walnut halves, finely chopped o 1 Medjool date, finely chopped o 20 g Red onion, diced o 1 Bird's eye chilli
- 40 g Rocket, to serve

INSTRUCTIONS
• Mix the yoghurt, lemon juice, coriander and spices together in a bowl. Add all the remaining ingredients and serve on a bed of the rocket.

INGREDIENTS:

- 2 ripe bananas o 250 ml milk o 2 tsp matcha green tea powder
- 1/2 tsp vanilla bean paste (not extract) or a small scrape of the seeds from a vanilla pod
- 6 ice cubes o 2 tsp honey

INSTRUCTIONS

- Simply blend all the ingredients together in a blender and serve in two glasses.

INGREDIENTS:

- o 50g rocket o 50g chicory leaves
- o 100g smoked salmon slices (you can also use lentils, cooked chicken breast or tinned tuna)
- o 80g avocado, peeled, stoned and sliced o 40g celery, sliced o 20g red onion, sliced o 15g walnuts, chopped
- o 1 tbs capers
- o 1 large Medjool date, pitted and chopped
- o 1 tbs extra-virgin olive oil
- o Juice ¼ lemon o 10g parsley, chopped
- o 10g lovage or celery leaves, chopped

INSTRUCTIONS

- Arrange the salad leaves on a large plate. Mix all the remaining ingredients together and serve on top of the leaves.

INGREDIENTS:

- 350ml milk o 150g buckwheat flour

- 1 large egg

- 1 tbsp extra virgin olive oil, for cooking

- For the chocolate sauce

- 100g dark chocolate (85 percent cocoa solids) o 85ml milk o 1 tbsp double cream o 1 tbsp extra virgin olive oil

To serve
o 400g strawberries, hulled and chopped o 100g walnuts, chopped

and blend until you have a smooth batter. It should not be too thick or too runny. (You can store any excess batter in an airtight container for up to 5 days in your fridge. Be sure to mix well before using again)

- To make the chocolate sauce, melt the chocolate in a heatproof bowl over a pan of simmering water. Once melted, mix in the milk, whisking thoroughly and then add the double cream and olive oil. You can keep the sauce warm by leaving the water in the pan simmering on a very low heat until your pancakes are ready.

- To make the pancakes heat a heavy-bottomed frying pan until it starts to smoke, then add the olive oil.

- Pour some of the batter into the centre of the pan, then tip the excess batter around it until you have covered the whole surface, you may have to add a little more batter to achieve this. You will only need to cook the pancake for 1

- Once you can see it going brown around the edges use a spatula to loosen the pancake around its edge, then flip it over. Try to flip in one action to avoid breaking it.

- Cook for a further minute or so on the other side and transfer to a plate.

- Place some strawberries in the centre and roll up the pancake. Continue until you have made as many pancakes as required.

- Spoon over a generous amount of sauce and sprinkle over some chopped walnuts.

INGREDIENTS:

For the Blueberry Banana Pancakes o 6 bananas o 6 eggs o 150g rolled oats o 2 tsp baking powder o ¼ teaspoon salt o 25g blueberries

For the Chunky Apple Compote o 2 apples o 5 dates (pitted) o 1 tablespoon lemon juice o 1/4 teaspoon cinnamon powder o pinch salt

INSTRUCTIONS
For the Blueberry Banana Pancakes

- Pop the rolled oats in a high-speed blender and pulse for 1 minute or until an oat flour has formed. Tip: make sure your blender is very dry before doing this or else everything will become soggy!

- Now add the bananas, eggs, baking powder and salt to the blender and pulse for 2 minutes until a smooth batter form.

the baking powder activates.

- To make your pancakes, add a dollop of butter (this helps to make them really delicious and crispy!) to your frying pan on a medium high heat. Add a few spoons of the blueberry pancake mix and fry for until nicely golden on the bottom side. Toss the pancake to fry the other side.

For the Chunky Apple Compote

- Core and rough chop your apples.

- Pop everything in a food processor, together with 2 tablespoons of water and a pinch of salt. Pulse to form your chunky apple compote.

INGREDIENTS:

For the Yoghurt Sauce o 1 cup
plain Greek yoghurt o 1 garlic
clove, minced o 1 to 2
tablespoons lemon juice
(from 1 lemon), to taste

- o ¼ teaspoon ground turmeric o 10 fresh mint leaves, minced o 2 teaspoons lemon zest (from 1 lemon)

For the Pancakes o 2 teaspoons ground turmeric o
1½ teaspoons ground cumin

- o 1 teaspoon salt o 1 teaspoon ground coriander o ½ teaspoon garlic powder
- o ½ teaspoon freshly ground black pepper o 1 head broccoli, cut into florets o 3 large eggs, lightly beaten
- o 2 tablespoons plain unsweetened almond milk
- o 1 cup almond flour o 4 teaspoons coconut oil

bowl. Taste and season with more lemon juice, if needed. Set aside or refrigerate until ready to serve.

- Make the pancakes. In a small bowl, combine the turmeric, cumin, salt, coriander, garlic and pepper.

- Place the broccoli in a food processor, and pulse until the florets are broken up into small pieces. Transfer the broccoli to a large bowl and add the eggs, almond milk, and almond flour. Stir in the spice mix and combine well.

- Heat 1 teaspoon of the coconut oil in a non-stick pan over medium-low heat. Pour ¼ cup batter into the skillet. Cook the pancake until small bubbles begin to appear on the surface and the bottom is golden brown, 2 to 3 minutes. Flip over and cook the pancake for 2 to 3 minutes more. To keep warm, transfer the cooked pancakes to an oven-safe dish and place in a 200°F oven.

- Continue making the remaining 3 pancakes, using the remaining oil and batter.

INGREDIENTS:

- o 1 cup buckwheat flour o 1/4 cup almond flour
- o 2 tablespoons hemp seeds, plus more for topping o 1 teaspoon baking powder o 1/2 teaspoon allspice o 1/4 teaspoon salt
- o 5.3 ounces pineapple Mauna cottage cheese o 1 egg
- o 2 tablespoons maple syrup, plus more for serving o 1 teaspoon vanilla extract
- o 1 cup unsweetened almond milk (or any other milk)
- o 1 small pineapple, outer layer cut off, sliced into rings and cored, (you can also use canned pineapple rings) o 1 tablespoon butter, divided

allspice and salt in a large bowl and whisk until combined.

- Add cottage cheese, egg, maple syrup, vanilla to the bowl. Whisk as you slowly add the milk until everything is well combined.

- Add a small bit of butter to the pan. Once melted, place one pineapple ring on top and cook until golden brown and starting to caramelize. Flip the pineapple slice over, spoon pancake batter on top so that it covers the ring entirely and spills over the sides a bit. Cook until set (about 3 minutes), carefully flip and cook another 2 minutes on the other side.

- Repeat with remaining pineapple rings and batter.

- Serve with maple syrup and extra hemp seeds for topping.

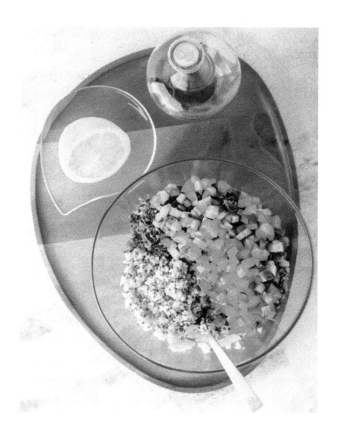

INGREDIENTS:

- 1 3/4 ounces (50g) arugula
- 1 3/4 ounces (50g) endive leaves
- 3 1/2 ounces (100g) smoked salmon slices
- 1/2 cup (80g) avocado, peeled, stoned, and sliced
- 1/2 cup (50g) celery including leaves, sliced
- 1/8 cup (20g) red onion, sliced
- 1/8 cups (15g) walnuts, chopped
- 1 tablespoon capers
- 1 large Medjool date, pitted and chopped
- 1 tablespoon extra-virgin olive oil
- juice of 1/4 lemon
- 1/4 cup (10g) parsley, chopped

INSTRUCTIONS:

- Place the salad leaves on a plate or in a large bowl.
- Mix all the remaining ingredients together and serve on top of the leaves.

INGREDIENTS:

- 1/3 pound (150g) shelled raw jumbo shrimp, deveined
- 2 teaspoons tamari (you can use soy sauce if you are not avoiding gluten)
- 2 teaspoons extra virgin olive oil
- 3 ounces (75g) soba (buckwheat noodles)
- 2 garlic cloves, finely chopped
- 1 Thai chili, finely chopped
- 1 teaspoon finely chopped fresh ginger
- 1/8 cup (20g) red onions, sliced
- 1/2 cup (45g) celery including leaves, trimmed and sliced, with leaves set aside
- 1/2 cup (75g) green beans, chopped
- 3/4 cup (50g) kale, roughly chopped
- 1/2 cup (100ml) chicken stock

shrimp in 1 teaspoon of the tamari and 1
teaspoon of the oil for 2 to 3 minutes.

- Transfer the shrimp to a plate. Wipe the pan out
  with a paper towel, as you're going to use it
  again.

- Cook the noodles in boiling water for 5 to 8
  minutes or as directed on the package. Drain
  and set aside.

- Meanwhile, fry the garlic, chili, ginger, red
  onion, celery (but not the leaves), green beans,
  and kale in the remaining tamari and oil over
  medium-high heat for 2 to 3 minutes. Add the
  stock and bring to a boil, then simmer for a
  minute or two, until the vegetables are cooked
  but still crunchy.

- Add the shrimp, noodles, and celery leaves to
  the pan, bring back to a boil, then remove from
  the heat and serve.

- 1/3 cup (50g) buckwheat
- 1 tablespoon ground turmeric
- 1/2 cup (80g) avocado
- 3/8 cup (65g) tomato
- 1/8 cup (20g) red onion
- 1/8 cup (25g) Medjool dates, pitted
- 1 tablespoon capers
- 3/4 cup (30g) parsley
- 2/3 cup (100g) strawberries, hulled
- 1 tablespoon extra-virgin olive oil
- juice of 1/2 lemon
- 1-ounce (30g) arugula

INSTRUCTIONS:

- Cook the buckwheat with the turmeric according to the package instructions.
- Drain and set aside to cool.
- Finely chop the avocado, tomato, red onion, dates, capers, and parsley and mix with the cool buckwheat.
- Slice the strawberries and gently mix into the salad with the oil and lemon juice. Serve on a bed of arugula.

- INGREDIENTS
- 125 g Lean minced beef (5% fat)
- 15 g Red onion, finely chopped
- 1 tsp. Parsley, finely chopped
- 1 tsp. Extra virgin olive oil
- 150 g Sweet potatoes
- 1 tsp. Extra virgin olive oil
- 1 tsp. Dried rosemary
- 1 Garlic clove, unpeeled
- 10 g Cheddar cheese, sliced or grated
- 150 g Red onion, sliced into rings
- 30 g Tomato, sliced
- 10 g Rocket
- 1 Gherkin (optional)

- Start by making the fries. Peel and cut the sweet potato into 1cm- thick chips. Toss them with the olive oil, rose- mary and garlic clove. Place on a baking sheet and roast for 30 minutes, until nice and crispy.
- For the burger, mix the onion and parsley with the minced beef. If you have pastry cutters, you could mould your burger with the largest pastry cutter in the set, otherwise, just use your hands to make a nice even patty.
- Heat a frying pan over a medium heat, add the olive oil, then place the burger on one side of the pan and the onion rings on the other. Cook the burger for 6 minutes on each side, ensuring it is cooked through. Fry the onion rings until cooked to your liking.
- When the burger is cooked, top it with the cheese and red onion and place it in the hot oven for a minute to melt the cheese. Remove and top with the tomato, rocket and gherkin. Serve with the fries.

- Raw or cooked prawns (Ideally king prawns)
- 65 g Buckwheat pasta
- 1 tbsp. Extra virgin olive oil
- 40 g Red onion, finely chopped
- 1 Garlic clove, finely chopped
- 30 g Celery, finely chopped
- 1 Bird's eye chilli, finely chopped
- 1 tsp. Dried mixed herbs
- 1 tsp. Extra virgin olive oil
- 2 tbsp. White wine (optional)
- 400 g Tinned chopped tomatoes
- 1 tbsp. Chopped parsley

herbs in the oil over a medium–low heat for 1–2 minutes. Turn the heat up to medium, add the wine and cook for 1 minute. Add the tomatoes and leave the sauce to simmer over a medium–low heat for 20–30 minutes, until it has a nice rich consistency. If you feel the sauce is getting too thick simply add a little water.

- While the sauce is cooking bring a pan of water to the boil and cook the pasta according to the packet instructions. When cooked to your liking, drain, toss with the olive oil and keep in the pan until needed.

- If you are using raw prawns add them to the sauce and cook for a further 3–4 minutes, until they have turned pink and opaque, add the parsley and serve. If you are using cooked prawns add them with the parsley, bring the sauce to the boil and serve.

- Add the cooked pasta to the sauce, mix thoroughly but gently and serve.

Ingredients:

- 60 g of broccoli only the flowers, without stems
- 75 g canned white beans
- 20 g red onion, thinly sliced
- 40 g canned artichokes cut into 4 pieces
- 15 g black olives
- 1 tablespoon chopped parsley
- ½ lemon (the juice)
- 1 teaspoon extra virgin olive oil
- 30 g of arugula
- 1 tablespoon roasted pumpkin seeds

Instructions:

- Chop the broccoli until it looks like couscous, by hand or with a blender.
- In a bowl, combine all other ingredients except arugula and squash seeds.
- In a plate, place the mixture on top of the arugula, sprinkle with the squash seeds. Serve

- Ingredients
- 65 g of buckwheat pasta
- 30 g red onion, thinly sliced
- 1 bird's eye pepper, finely chopped
- 30 g of finely chopped celery
- 30 g rapped carrots
- 75 g peeled beans
- For seasoning
- 1-2 cm fresh ginger
- ¼ of lime (the juice)
- 1 tsp. tamarind or soy sauce
- 2 teaspoons of olive oil
- 1 tablespoon chopped cilantro
- 1 teaspoon sesame seeds

Instructions
- Cook the buckwheat pasta as indicated on the package, drain and rinse with cold water. Leave to cool.

Ingredients

- 60 g of buckwheat pasta
- 50 g canned artichokes (oil or water) drained and cut into pieces
- 1 tomato (130 g) cut into 8 pieces
- 1 teaspoon of capers
- 10 g red onion, thinly sliced
- 1 teaspoon extra virgin olive oil
- ½ lemon (the juice)
- 1 tablespoon chopped parsley
- 2 slices of Parma ham (or other cured ham)
- 20 g of arugula
- 15 g Parmesan (or other Italian cheese)

Instructions

- Cook the buckwheat pasta as indicated on the package. Drain and set aside.
- In a bowl, mix artichokes, tomato, capers, red onion, olive oil, lemon juice and parsley.
- Add the pasta mixture.
- Cut the ham into strips and mix with the pasta.
- Arrange the arugula on a plate. Place the pasta, sprinkle with grated Parmesan cheese and serve.

Ingredients:

- 170 g/ 6 oz buckwheat groats
- 325 ml/ 11 fl.oz vegetable broth
- 2 tablespoons olive oil
- 2 garlic cloves
- 1 ½ tablespoons brown sugar, more to taste
- juice of 1 lemon, more to taste
- ½ teaspoons red chili flakes, more or less to taste
- ¼ teaspoon ground cumin
- ¼ teaspoon ground coriander
- 2 medium carrots, about 150 g/ 5.3 oz
- 3 medium scallions
- 1 bunch of parsley, about 20 g/ 0.7 oz
- fine sea salt and black pepper

- Bring the vegetable broth to a boil. Add the rinsed buckwheat groats, cover the saucepan with a tight-fitting lid and simmer on low heat until the buckwheat is done to your liking, more or less 10 minutes. Check the buckwheat's package instructions regarding the cooking times, they can differ from pack to pack and sometimes a lot. Check the buckwheat 2-3 minutes earlier than indicated on the package, just to make sure you don't overcook it. It should be soft, but still have a good bite. Mushy buckwheat is not good.
- Drain the buckwheat well, if there is still liquid left in the pan. Give the buckwheat to a large bowl and leave to cool.

olive oil, brown sugar, about ¾ of the freshly squeezed lemon juice, chili flakes, ground cumin, ground coriander, some salt and pepper. Stir well. Adjust the taste with more sugar, lemon juice and salt, if necessary. The dressing should taste sweet and very lemony, the flavours should be strong.

- Grate the carrots on the large holes of a greater box. Cut the scallions into fine rings. Chop the parsley, including most of the stems (only discard the lower thicker parts of the stems). Give the vegetables and the parsley to the buckwheat bowl.
- Pour the dressing over the salad and stir well. Adjust the taste again. Serve immediately or refrigerate until serving.
- Serve as suggested above.

Ingredients:

- 6 ounces whole-wheat penne pasta
- 2 large red bell peppers, chopped
- Zest of ½ lemon, grated
- Juice of 2 lemons
- 2 shallots, minced

Instructions:

- Follow the directions on the package and cook the pasta
- Place a pan over medium flame. Add rapeseed oil. Once the oil is heated, add red bell pepper and cook covered for 4-5 minutes or until slightly tender
- Move the red peppers from the pan to a plate and add salmon into the pan. Cook covered for 7-8 minutes or until the salmon flakes easily when pierced with a fork
- Meanwhile, add lemon juice, lemon zest, garlic, capers, shallot and olives into a large bowl and mix well
- Add pasta, salmon and red pepper and toss well. Sprinkle pepper on top. Drizzle oil. Toss well
- Cover and set aside until use
- Add rocket just before serving. Toss well and serve

Ingredients:

For the salad:

- 2 slice turkey bacon
- ½ avocado, peeled, pitted, diced
- ½ can (from 15 ounces can) water packed artichoke heart quarters, drained
- 1 bunch kale, discard hard stem and ribs, leaves thinly sliced
- ½ cup halved grape or cherry tomatoes
- 8 ounces cooked chicken, diced
- ½ cup sliced strawberries
- 2 hardboiled eggs, peeled, quartered lengthwise
- ½ cup crumbled goat cheese

- 1 finely chopped tablespoon Italian parsley
- 1 Small clove garlic, peeled, minced
- Pepper to taste
- 1 tablespoon fresh lemon juice
- ½ tablespoon Dijon mustard
- Salt to taste (optional)
- 2 scallions, thinly sliced, to garnish

Lay the bacon strips on the baking sheet

- Bake the bacon in an oven preheated to 350°F until brown and crisp, about 18-20 minutes, flipping sides halfway through baking
- When cool enough to handle, chop into small pieces and set aside
- To make the dressing: Add mayonnaise, parsley, garlic, pepper, lemon juice, mustard and salt into a bowl. Whisk well. Cover and set aside for a while for the flavours set in
- Divide the kale leaves onto 2 serving plates
- Layers with equal quantities of avocado, artichoke hearts, tomatoes, bacon, strawberries and chicken in any manner you desire
- Sprinkle scallions on top. Place 4 slices of egg on the salad. Scatter goat cheese on top
- Divide the dressing into 2 small bowls
- Serve the dressing on the side

Ingredients:

- **1** tablespoon minced shallot
- Salt to taste
- 1/4 cup extra-virgin olive oil
- 2 ounces oyster mushrooms, sliced
- ½ Belgian endive, cut into 1-inch pieces
- ½ small head escarole, use the inner pale coloured leaves only, chopped into 1-inch pieces
- 1/4 cup shaved Parmesan cheese
- 1 tablespoon sherry vinegar
- Freshly ground pepper to taste
- 2 ounces shiitake mushrooms, cut into thick slices
- 1 spring thyme
- ½ small head radicchio
- 2 tablespoons chopped flat-leaf parsley

pepper into a bowl and whisk well. Let it rest for 10 minutes
- Add 3 tablespoons oil and whisk well. Cover and set aside
- Place a skillet over medium flame. Add a tablespoon of oil. When the oil is heated, add mushrooms, salt, pepper and thyme cook until brown. Stir occasionally
- Transfer the mushrooms into a bowl. Throw off the thyme.
- Pour dressing over the mushrooms and toss well
- Add endive, escarole, radicchio and parsley and toss well. Taste and add more salt pepper if required
- Scatter cheese and toss well
- Serve

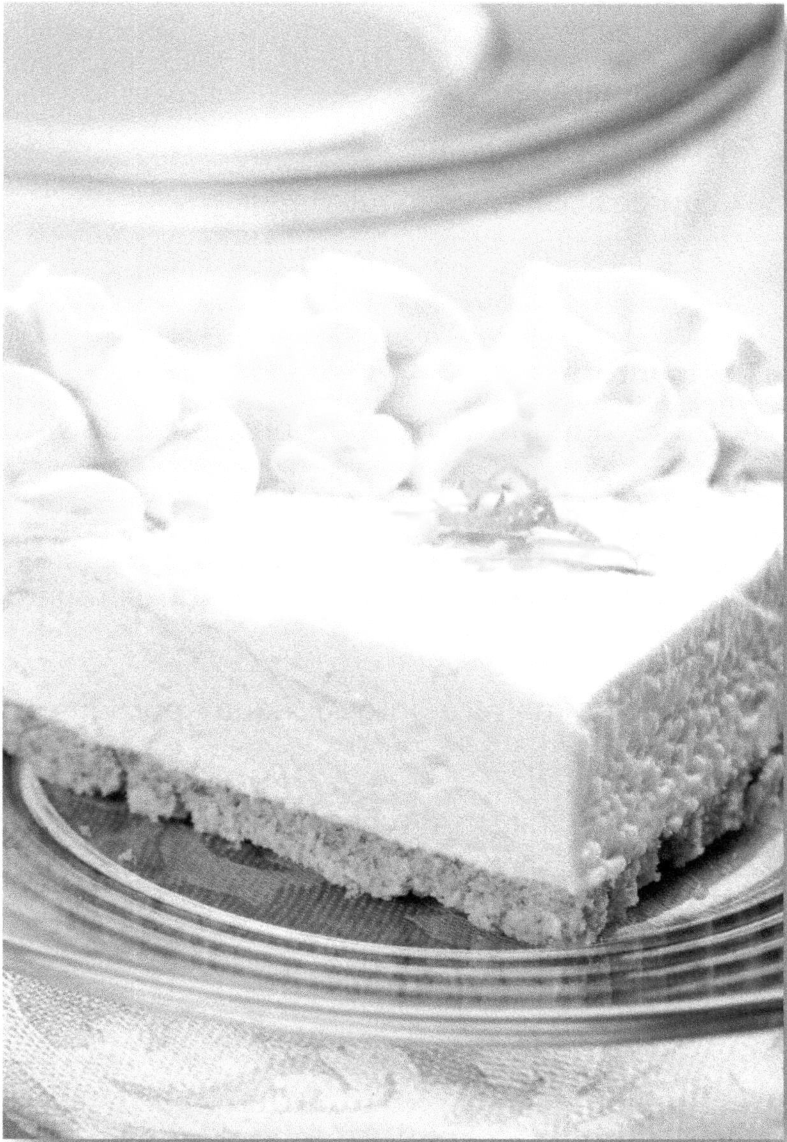

Ingredients:

- ¼ cup cashews
- ¼ cup almonds
- Zest of 1 ½ key limes
- ¾ cup desiccated coconut

Instructions:

- Add the nuts into the food processor bowl and give short pulses until finely chopped
- Add dates, lime juice and lime zest and pulse until well combined and the mixture sticks together when pressed
- Divide the mixture into 6 equal portions and shape into balls
- Dredge the bites in coconut and place in an airtight container. Refrigerate until use. It can last for a week

Ingredients:

- 2 packages (8 ounces each) cream cheese
- ¼ cup chopped fresh parsley
- 4 teaspoons mixed dried herbs (mixture of parsley, rosemary and thyme)
- ¼-½ cup crumbled blue cheese
- 4 teaspoons dried thyme, to garnish
- Assorted crackers to serve (optional)
- 2 tablespoons finely chopped walnuts

Instructions:

- Add cream cheese and blue cheese into a mixing bowl and set aside to soften for about 45 minutes
- Beat on low speed with an electric hand mixer until smooth, light and creamy
- Add dried herbs and parsley and mix well
- Cover the bowl with plastic wrap and chill 3-4 hours or until be shaped into a ball
- Shape the cheese mixture into one big ball. Place thyme and walnuts a plate and Stir. Dredge the ball in thyme mixture
- Cover and chill for at least a couple of hours
- Slice and serve as it is or with crackers

Ingredients:

- 4 blocks firm or extra-firm tofu,
- 4 tablespoons soy sauce
- 2 cups breadcrumbs
- 2 teaspoons lemon pepper
- ½ cup soy milk
- 4 tablespoons crumbled nori seaweed
- Flour, as required
- Salt to taste

Instructions:

- To press tofu: Place tofu over layers of paper towels. Place more towels on top of the tofu
- Place something heavy over the tofu. Let it remain like this for 20 minutes. Cut tofu into strips like sticks
- Prepare a baking sheet by lining it with parchment paper
- Place breadcrumbs in a shallow bowl
- Dredge tofu in flour and place on a tray
- Combine soy milk, salt, lemon juice and soy sauce in a 2nd shallow bowl
- Combine breadcrumbs, lemon pepper and nori in a 3rd shallow bowl
- Dunk tofu in soymilk mixture, one at a time. Shake off excess milk mixture and dredge it in breadcrumbs mixture and place on the baking sheet
- Bake tofu in an oven preheated to 375°F, for about 45 minutes or until crisp and brown

Ingredients:

- 7 ounces pitted dates
- 3 tablespoons cocoa
- ½ teaspoon ground cinnamon
- ½ desiccated coconut
- 1/3 cup roasted almonds
- 1 teaspoon vanilla extract

To garnish:

- 15 roasted almonds

Instructions:

- Add dates, cocoa, cinnamon, coconut, almonds and vanilla into the food processor bowl and blend until well combined
- Divide the mixture into 15 equal portions and shape into balls
- Place an almond on each ball and press to adhere and flatten the ball
- Place in an airtight container and refrigerate until use. It can last 15 days

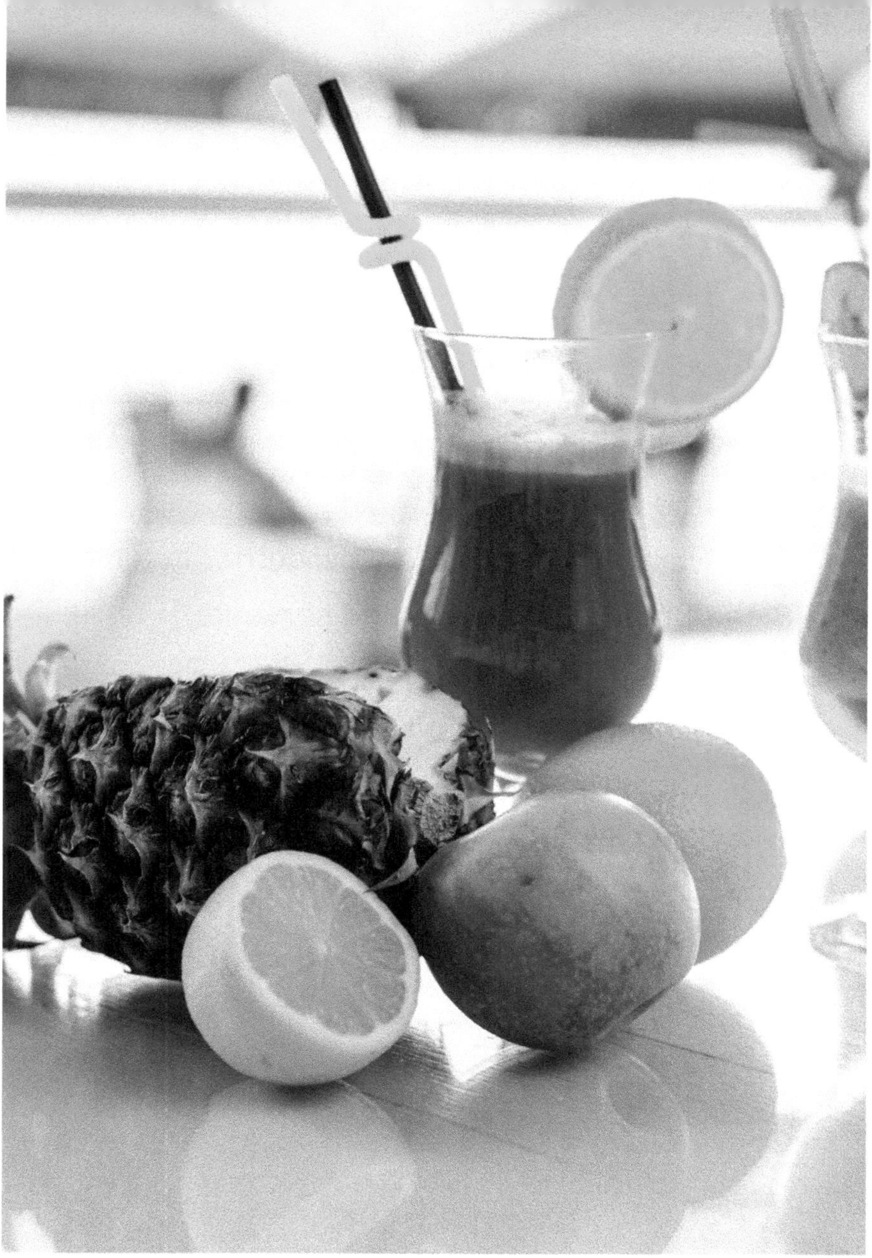

INGREDIENTS:

- 2 tsp honey
- 1 cup freshly made green tea
- 10 baby kale leaves, stalks removed
- 1 ripe banana
- 6 ice cubes

INSTRUCTIONS:

- First of all, stir the honey into the warm green tea until it is dissolved
- Now whiz all the ingredients together in a blender
- Blend until gets smooth and serve it

INGREDIENTS:
- ½ heaped tsp turmeric powder
- ½ tablespoon fresh ginger, grated
- 1 small lemon
- Orange zest
- 1 teaspoon honey

INSTRUCTIONS:
- Boil 200ml of water in the kettle
- Place the turmeric, ginger, and orange zest in a teapot, pour over the boiling water and let stand for 5 minutes
- Drain through a tea strainer into a cup, add lemon juice or slice of lemon sweeten with honey

INGREDIENTS:
- 5 ounces parsley, stem and leaves
- 2 teaspoons honey
- 2 green apples, cored, sliced
- A handful fresh mint leaves
- 2 inches ginger, sliced

INSTRUCTIONS:
- Add parsley, ginger, apples and mint leaves into a juicer and extract the juice
- Add honey and stir
- Pour into glasses and serve

- 2 inches fresh ginger, sliced
- 2 cucumber, trimmed, chopped
- Juice of lime
- 2 cups coconut water
- 2 cups baby kale leaves
- 2 very large chard leaves, torn
- 2 stalks celery, chopped
- 2 apples, cored, sliced
- 2 cups packed arugula

INSTRUCTIONS:
- Squeeze out juice from lime and lemon
- Add apples, ginger, kale, chard, arugula, and cucumber and extra the juice
- Stir in the coconut water, lime and lemon juice
- Pour into 2 glasses
- Add ice if desired and serve right away

Savoury Kale and Tomato Juice

INGREDIENTS:

- 6 medium plum tomatoes, chopped into chunks
- 4 stalks celery, chopped
- Juice of large lemon
- 2 cups flat-leaf parsley
- 2 tablespoons chia seed (optional)

INSTRUCTIONS:

- Add tomatoes and parsley into the juicer first followed by celery and kale. Extract the juice and stir in the lemon juice and chia seeds
- Let it rest for 5 minutes
- Pour into 2 glasses and serve

INGREDIENTS:

- 4 tablespoons vanilla soy milk or any other milk of your choice
- Stevia to taste
- 4 tablespoons coconut oil
- 2 cups brewed coffee

INSTRUCTIONS:

- Add coffee, coconut oil, milk and stevia into a blender
- Blend until well combined and frothy. It can take a couple of minutes. You can also make it in a frothier
- Pour into mugs and serve

Coconut Oil Hot Chocolate

INGREDIENTS:
- 1 cup full-fat coconut milk
- 1 cup filtered water
- 4 tablespoons grass-fed butter, unsalted
- 4 tablespoons raw cacao powder or cocoa powder
- 1/ teaspoon ground cinnamon or taste 2 tablespoons coconut oil
- ½ teaspoon vanilla extract

INSTRUCTIONS:
- Add water and coconut milk into a saucepan. Place the saucepan over medium flame
- When the mixture comes to boil, turn off the heat

- ½ teaspoon ground cinnamon
- A pinch black pepper
- A pinch cayenne peppers
- ½ teaspoon turmeric powder
- ½ teaspoon raw honey
- 2 slices, peeled ginger

INSTRUCTIONS:
- Blend milk, honey, ginger and all the spices in a blender until smooth
- Transfer into a saucepan. Place the saucepan over medium flame and heat for about 3 minutes, until hot, making sure not to boil it
- Pour into a mug and serve

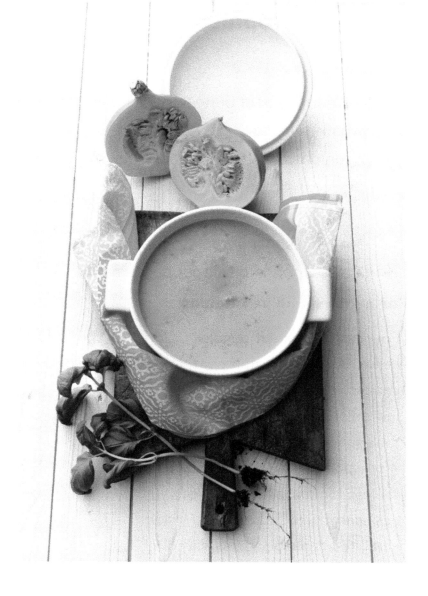

Noodles

Ingredients:

For bone broth:

- 6.6 pounds beef bones or chicken carcasses or lamb bones
- 2 onions or leeks or carrots or celery, chopped into chunks
- 4 bay leaves
- 3-4 tablespoons apple cider vinegar
- 2 tablespoons black peppercorns

For noodles and vegetables:

- 24 ounces buckwheat noodles
- 8 heads Bok Choy, trimmed, thinly sliced
- 2 carrots, cut into matchsticks
- 4 inches piece fresh ginger root, peeled, grated
- 8 tablespoons lime juice
- 3-4 teaspoons tamari or soy sauce
- 2 tablespoon extra-virgin olive oil
- 14 ounces mixed mushrooms, sliced
- 1 small red cabbage, thinly sliced
- 12 spring onions, thinly sliced diagonally
- 4 tablespoons miso paste
- 1 cup chopped fresh cilantro

cider vinegar, and peppercorns into a large stock pot. Cover with enough water, such that the water level is about 3 inches above the bones
- Place the pot over high flame. When it comes to a boil, lower the heat and cook covered, for 6 hours if you are using chicken or about 12 hours if you are using beef bones or lamb bones
- Remove any scrum that floats on top, time to time
- Place a strainer over a jar and strain the broth. The broth is ready to use
- To make noodles: Follow the directions on the package and cook the buckwheat noodles
- Drizzle oil over the strained and rinsed noodles. Toss well
- Pour 8 cups of broth into stock pot. Store the remaining broth in the refrigerator and use it in some other recipes. If your broth is hot, proceed to the next step else heat up the broth
- Add ginger, lime juice, tamari, miso and spring onions into the stock pot and mix well
- Place equal quantities of Bok Choy, carrots, mushrooms and red cabbage into 8 soup bowl
- Pour a cup of broth into each cup. Divide the noodles among the bowls
- Garnish with cilantro and serve

Ingredients:

- 2 ½ cups ripe, peeled, seeded, cubed cantaloupe
- 2/3 cup fresh orange juice
- 1 ½ tablespoons fresh lime or lemon juice
- ½ cup ripe strawberries, hulled
- ¼ cup dry red wine
- 10-20 fresh mint leaves
- Stevia to taste (optional)

To serve:

- Sliced strawberries
- Mint leaves for

Instructions:

- Add cantaloupe and strawberries into a blender and blitz smooth
- Add orange juice, wine and lime juice and blend until smooth. Transfer into a bowl
- Add mint. Mix well. Add stevia if using. Mix well
- Cover the bowl with cling wrap and refrigerate for 3-4 hours
- Ladle into soup bowl. Garnish with sliced strawberries and mint leaves and serve

Ingredients:

- ½ tablespoon extra-virgin olive oil
- ¾ cup sliced white mushrooms
- 2 cloves garlic, peeled, minced
- 2 cups vegetable broth
- ½ can (from 15 ounces can) tomato sauce
- ½ teaspoon kosher salt
- Crushed red pepper to taste
- Black pepper powder to taste
- ½ teaspoon dried basil
- 6 tablespoons grated parmesan cheese
- ¼ cup diced red onions
- 1 small zucchini, diced
- 2 tablespoons dry red wine
- ½ can (from 14.5 ounces can) petite diced tomatoes
- ½ tablespoon Italian seasoning
- ¼ teaspoon garlic salt
- 1 cup buckwheat noodles
- A handful fresh parsley, chopped, to garnish

mushrooms and sauté for 2-3 minutes

- Stir in the zucchini and sauté for a couple of minutes. Add wine and stir.
- When the mixture begins to boil, add broth, tomato sauce, diced tomatoes, basil, salt and spices
- Once it stars boiling, lower heat to medium low and stir in the buckwheat noodles. Cook until the noodles are al dente. Remove from heat and add Parmesan cheese. Stir
- Ladle into soup bowls. Garnish with parsley and serve

Ingredients:

- 1pound beef shank with bone
- 1 teaspoon salt or to taste
- ½ medium red onion, chopped + extra finely chopped, to garnish
- 1 bird's eye chili, sliced
- 2 cups water
- 1 ½ cups beef broth
- 1 medium carrot, peeled, coarsely chopped
- 1 small potato, quartered
- 1 chayote, peeled, chopped into chucks
- 1/8 cup sliced pickled jalapenos
- ½ cup chopped, fresh cilantro, divide
- 2 radishes, quartered + extra to serve
- ½ tablespoon olive oil
- 1 tablespoon black pepper or to taste
- ½ can (from 14.5 ounce can) diced tomatoes
- 1 ear corn, husked, cut unto thirds
- 1 small head cabbage, cored, cut into wedges
- Lime juice to taste

- Place a heavy soup pot or any other heavy pot like a Dutch oven over medium flame. Add oil and swirl the pot so the oil spreads all over the bottom of the pot
- Once oil is heated, add meat, bones, salt and pepper and mix well
- Once it turns brown, add chopped onions and cook until the onions are light brown, stirring frequently. Add tomatoes and broth. The broth should cover the bones. If the broth is not covering the bones, pour some water to keep it covered
- When it comes to a boil, lower the heat and cover the pot loosely with a lid. Simmer until the meat is tender
- Add remaining water and continue simmering. Add carrots, bird's eye chili, half the cilantro, potatoes, chayote and corn. Cook until the potatoes and chayote are tender
- Add the cabbage and simmer for another 10 minutes. Turn off the heat
- Ladle into soup bowls. Garnish with jalapenos, finely chopped onions and the remaining cilantro over it
- Pour some lime juice into each bowl and top with radishes

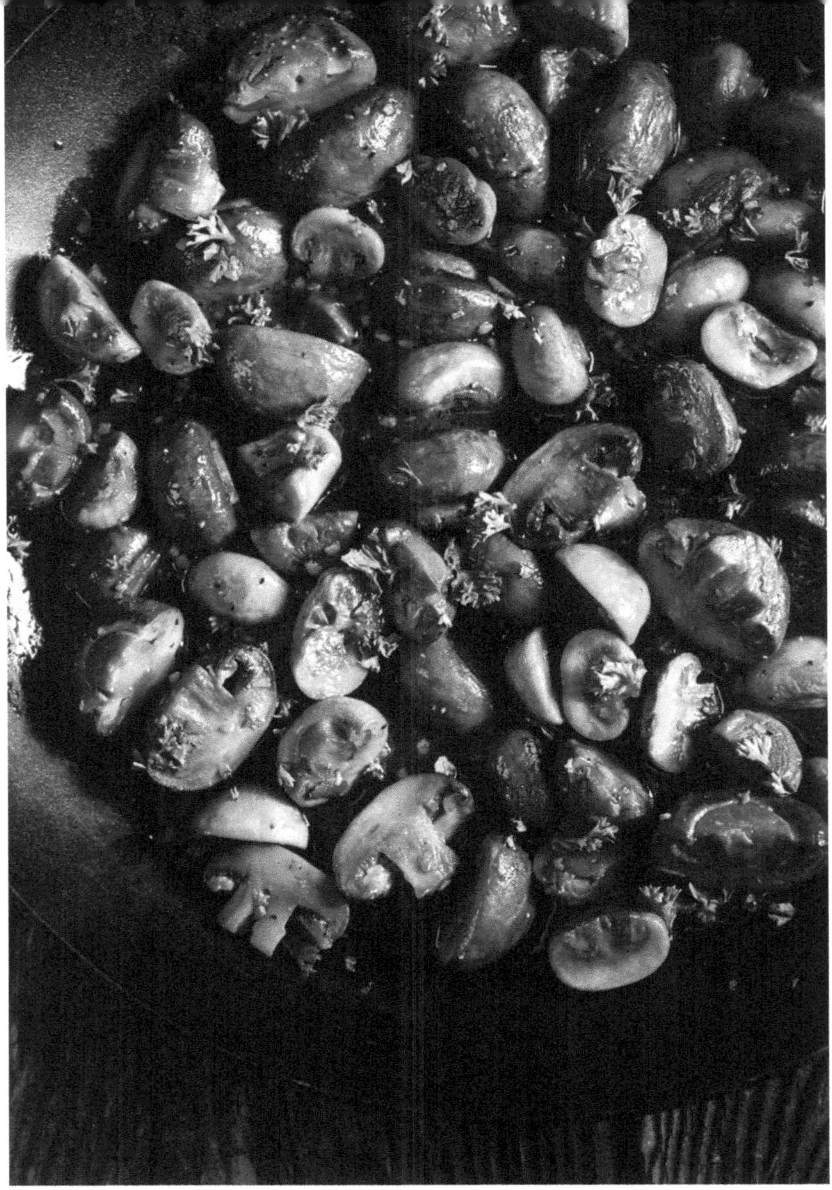

Ingredients:

For walnut mayonnaise:

- 2 tablespoons finely chopped walnuts
- 3-4 tablespoons mayonnaise
- ½ tablespoon chopped, fresh parsley

For walnut mayonnaise:

- 4 slices whole-wheat bread
- ½ green apple, peeled, cored, cut into thin slices
- Cooked, sliced turkey, as required
- A handful rockets

Instructions:

- To make walnut mayonnaise: Combine walnuts, mayonnaise, mustard and parsley in a bowl
- Smear walnut mayonnaise on one side if the bread slices
- Place arugula on 2 bread slices, on the mayo side. Place turkey slices over it followed by apple slices
- Complete the sandwich by covering with remaining bread slices, with mayo side facing down
- Cut into desired shape and serve

Ingredients:

- ½ pound lean ground turkey
- ½ cup chopped yellow or red onion
- Pepper to taste
- 1 teaspoon olive oil
- 1 jalapeno or taste, chopped
- ½ tablespoon minced garlic
- ¼ teaspoon ground cumin
- 2 teaspoons red pepper flakes
- ½ cup chopped fresh cilantro
- Salt to taste
- A handful parsley leaves

Instructions:

- Place a skillet over medium flame. Add oil and wait for it to heat. Add garlic and sauté for about a minute until light brown
- Stir in onions, tomatoes, jalapeno, parsley and red peer flakes and cook for 4-5 minutes
- Stir in the turkey and cook until brown, breaking the turkey as it cooks
- Add cilantro, salt and pepper and stir
- Serve hot

Ingredients:
- Pound sirloin steak
- ¼ teaspoon pepper or taste
- ¼ teaspoon garlic powder
- Salt to taste
- ¼ teaspoon ground cumin

For chimichurri sauce:
- A handful fresh parsley, finely chopped
- Tablespoon finely chopped shallot
- A handful kale and spring mix, finely chopped
- ¼ cup olive oil
- 1/8 teaspoon salt or taste
- Cloves garlic, peeled, minced
- ½ teaspoon honey
- ¼ teaspoon crushed red pepper flakes

salt, honey and red pepper flakes into a bowl
and mix well. Cover and set aside for a few
minutes

- Meanwhile, set up your grill and preheat it to
medium-high
- Sprinkle salt and spices all over the steak and
rub it well into it
- Place the steak on the grill and cook for 8
minutes. Flip the steak and cook for 8 minutes
for medium- rare or to the desired doneness
- Remove the steak from the grill and cover with
foil and let it sit for 15 minutes
- Cut into slices and divide into plate. Spread
chimichurri sauce on top and serve

Ingredients:
- 7 ounces potatoes, peeled, cut into 1inch cubes
- A handful fresh parsley, chopped
- ½ ounce kale leaves, chopped, discard hard stems and ribs
- 2 beef fillet steaks (4-5 ounces each) or 1inch thick sirloin steak
- ¼ cup beef stock
- Salt to taste
- ½ teaspoons corn-starch mixed with 2 tablespoons water
- ½ tablespoon extra-virgin olive oil
- Medium red onion, cut into thin rings
- Cloves garlic, finely chopped
- Pepper to taste
- Tablespoons red wine
- 2 teaspoons tomato puree

4 minutes. Drain in a colander
- Transfer the potatoes into baking dish. Drizzle a tablespoon of oil over the potatoes and toss well. Spread it evenly
- Bake in an oven preheated to 440°F, for about 30-40 minutes. Stir the potatoes at intervals of 10 minutes
- Transfer into a bowl. Add parsley and toss well
- Place a skillet over medium flame. Add ½ tablespoon oil. When the oil is heated, add onion and cook until golden brown. Transfer into a bowl
- Steam kale in the streaming equipment you have
- Add ½ tablespoon oil into the skillet. Add garlic and cook for few seconds until fragrant. Stir in the kale and cook for a couple of minutes, until is turns slightly limp. Turn off the heat. Cover and set aside
- Place on ovenproof pan over high-high flame. Add remaining oil and wait for the oil to heat. Once the oil is heated, add steaks and coat it with oil, on both the sides. Cook for 3 to 4 minutes on each side. Turn off the heat
- Shift the saucepan into an oven preheated to 440°F, and roast until the meat is cooked to desired doneness
- Take out the pan from the over. Set the meat aside on a plate

Ingredients:

- ½ pound Orecchiette
- ½ pound sweet Italian sausage, discard casings
- ¼ teaspoon crushed red pepper
- Salt to taste
- 2 tablespoons grated pecorino+ extra to garnish
- 2 tablespoons extra-virgin olive oil
- 1 clove garlic, peeled, thinly sliced
- ½ pound chicory or escarole chopped
- ½ cup chicken stock
- A handful fresh mint leaves, chopped

- Place a large skillet over medium flame. Add a tablespoon of oil and let it heat
- Once oil heated, add sausage and cook until brown. Break it while it cooks
- Remove sausage with a slotted spoon and place on a plate
- Add a tablespoon of oil. When the oil is heated, add garlic and red pepper and stir for few seconds until you get a nice aroma
- Stir in chicory and salt and cook covered, until they turn limp. It should take a couple of minutes
- Uncover and continue cooking until tender
- Add pasta, sausage, cheese and stock and cook until the sauce is slightly thick. Add mint and stir
- Serve hot

Ingredients:
- 4 tablespoons olive oil
- 2 inches ginger, peeled, grated
- 2 teaspoons chili flakes
- 2 sticks cinnamon
- 3.5 pounds lamb neck fillet, cut into bite size pieces
- 7 ounces medjool dates, pitted, chopped
- 2.2 pounds butternut squash, cut into ½ inch cubes
- A handful fresh cilantro, chopped+ extra to serve
- 2 red onions, sliced
- 6 cloves garlic grated
- 4 teaspoons cumin seeds
- 4 teaspoons turmeric powder
- Salt to taste
- 2 cans (14 ounces each) chopped tomatoes
- 1 can water
- 2 cans (14.1 ounces each) chickpeas, drained

To serve:
- Cooked buckwheat
- Couscous
- Rice
- Flatbreads

oven, over medium flame. Add 4 tablespoons of oil and wait for it to heat. Once oil is heated, add onion and cook covered until it softens
- Stir in the ginger, garlic and all the spices. Cook for a few seconds until aromatic. Add 2-3 tablespoons of water if the spices are getting burnt
- Stir in the lamb. Stir until the lamb is well coated with the spice mixture
- Add dates, tomatoes and water and mix well. When it comes to a boil, turn off the heat
- Cover the pot and shift the pan into an oven preheated to 440°F, and bake for about 80-90 minutes or until lamb is well-cooked. Add butternut squash and chickpeas during the last 30 minutes of cooking
- Add cilantro and stir
- Serve with any one of serving options

Ingredients:

- ¾ pound lean ground lamb
- 1 clove garlic, minced
- ½ cup dry red wine
- 1 teaspoon ground cumin
- Salt to taste
- Hot sauce to taste (optional)
- ½ cup chopped red onion
- 1 can (14.1 ounces) whole tomatoes, with its liquid, chopped
- ½ tablespoons chili powder
- 1 teaspoon dried oregano
- 1 ½ cans (15 ounces each) black beans, drained
- ½ teaspoons sugar
- Fresh cilantro springs (optional)

Break it while you stir

- Remove the mixture with a slotted spoon and place on a plate lied with paper towels. Discard the fat remaining in the pan. Wipe the pot clean
- Place the pot, spices, oregano and salt and stir. Heat thoroughly
- Lower the heat and cook covered, for an hour. Add beans and hot sauce and stir
- Cover and simmer for about 30 minutes
- Sprinkle cilantro on top and serve

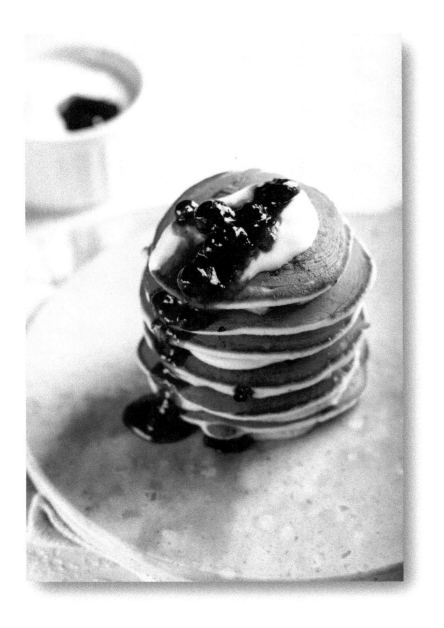

INGREDIENTS:
- 75g porridge oats
- 125g plain flour
- 2 tbsp caster sugar
- Pinch of salt
- 2 apples, peeled, cored and cut into small pieces
- 300ml semi-skimmed mild
- 2 egg whites
- 2 tsp light olive oil

For the compote:
- 120g blackcurrants, washed and stalks removed
- 2 tbsp caster sugar
- 3 tbsp water

simmer and cook for 10-15 minutes.

- Place the oats, flour, baking powder, caster sugar and salt in a large bowl and mix well. Stir in the apple and then whisk in the milk a little at a time until you have a smooth mixture. Whisk the egg whites to stiff peaks and then fold into the pancake batter. Transfer the batter to a jug.
- Heat 1/2 tsp oil in a non-stick frying pan on a medium-high heat and pour in approximately one quarter of the batter. Cook on both sides until golden brown. Remove and repeat to make four pancakes.
- Serve the pancakes with the blackcurrant compote drizzled over.

Mocha Chocolate Mousse-New Sirtfood Recipes

INGREDIENTS:

- 250g dark chocolate (85% cocoa solids)
- 6 medium free-range eggs, separated
- 4 tbsp strong black coffee
- 4 tbsp almond milk
- Chocolate coffee beans, to decorate

INSTRUCTIONS:

- Melt the chocolate in a large bowl set over a pan of gently simmering water, making sure the bottom of the bowl doesn't touch the water. Remove the bowl from the heat and leave the melted chocolate to cool to room temperature.
- Once the melted chocolate is at room temperature, whisk in the egg yolks one at a time and then gently fold in the coffee and almond milk.

- Using a hand-held electric mixer, whisk the egg whites until stiff peaks form, then mix a couple of tablespoons into the chocolate mixture to loosen it. Gently fold in the remainder, using a large metal spoon.

- Transfer the mousse to individual glasses and smooth the surface. Cover with cling film and chill for at least 2 hours, ideally overnight. Decorate with chocolate coffee beans before serving.

Ingredients:

- 4 cups whole-wheat pastry flour
- 1 teaspoon baking soda
- 3 teaspoons double-acting baking powder
- ½ cup arrowroot starch
- ½ teaspoon salt
- 8 large eggs
- 2 tablespoons vanilla extra
- 2 teaspoons almond extra
- 2/3 cup vanilla whey protein powder
- 1 cup plain, non-fat Greek yogurt
- 1 ½ cups unsweetened applesauce
- 4 teaspoons liquid stevia
- 1 cup granulated erythritol
- 4 tablespoons matcha powder
  For frosting:
- 3 cups fat-free cottage cheese
- 2 teaspoons vanilla paste
- 1 teaspoon almond extra
- 4 tablespoons matcha powder
- 8 ounces Neuchatel cream cheese, softened
- 2 teaspoons liquid stevia
- 2 cups vanilla whey protein powder

it with parchment paper

- Add whole-wheat flour, baking powder, arrowroot, salt and baking soda into a bowl and stir well
- Add eggs, yogurt, applesauce, stevia, vanilla and almond extract into another bowl and whisk until well incorporated
- Add protein powder, erythritol and matcha powder and continue whisking until well incorporate and free from lumps
- Add the flour mixture and continue whisking until just combined, making sure not to over-mix
- Divide the batter among the prepared baking pans
- Bake the cakes in an oven preheated to 325°F, for about 30-35 minutes or until firm on top. When the cakes are ready, if you press the top of the cupcake, it should spring back
- Cool the cakes on your countertop. Invert the cakes on plates and peel off the parchment paper
- Place on cake on a cake stand

texture. You can also blend it using an electric hand mixer

- Blend in the vanilla, almond extract and stevia
- Next goes in the protein powder and mathca powder and blitz until smooth
- Spread some of the frosting on the cake (the one on the cake stand). Carefully place the other cake over the frosted cake. Spread frosting on top and sides of the cake
- Chill for a couple of hours
- Slice and serve

Ingredients:

- 8.8 ounces compound dark chocolate
- 2 cups brown sugar
- ½ cup cocoa powder
- 4 eggs
- 1 cup chopped walnuts
- 5.3 ounces butter
- 1 ½ cups buckwheat flour
- 1 teaspoon baking powder
- ½ cup warm milk, if needed
- 4 tablespoons cacao nibs
- 2 teaspoons whole wheat flour

- Add chocolate and butter into a microwave safe container and melt the mixture in microwave. Stir every 15 seconds until it melts
- Add eggs into a bowl and whisk well. Whisk in sugar, ¼ cup at a time and beat well each time
- Pour melted chocolate and whisk until well combined
- Combine cocoa, baking powder and buckwheat flour in a bowl. Add the mixture of dry ingredients into the bowl of chocolate mixture, a tablespoon at time and fold gently each time
- Spoon the batter into the baking pan
- Combine cacao nibs and walnut mixture over the butter and swirl lightly
- Bake the brownies in an over preheated to 300°F, four about 10 minutes or until firm on top. It will be slightly sticky in the middle
- Cool to room temperature. Cut into 12 equal squares and serve
- Store leftovers in an aright container in the refrigerator. It can last for 4-5 days

Vegan Buckwheat Chocolate Chip Cookies

Ingredients:

- 2 cups buckwheat flour
- 2/3 cup melted coconut oil
- 2 teaspoons vanilla extract
- 1 teaspoon baking soda
- 1 cup dark chocolate chips
- 1 cup coconut sugar
- 4 tablespoons water
- 1 tablespoon fine sea salt
- 2 teaspoons apple cider vinegar

- Combine buckwheat flour, oil, vanilla, baking soda, coconut sugar, water and salt in a bowl
- Add vinegar and ix well. Add chocolate chips and fold gently
- Divide the dough into 24 equal portions and place on the baking sheets. Leave sufficient gap between the cookies. Press lightly to flatten
- Bake to the cookies in an oven preheated to 350°F, for about 10 minutes or until firm around the edges
- Let the cookies cool on the baking sheet for 10 minutes. Remove the cookies from the biking sheet and place on wire rack to cool
- Once completely cooled, place the cookies in an airtight container. It can last for about 4-5 days

Ingredients:

- 3 tablespoons unsalted butter
- ¼ cup buckwheat flour
- ¼ teaspoon + 1/8 teaspoon baking powder
- ¼ cup + 1 tablespoon cane sugar
- ½ teaspoon vanilla extract
- 6 ounces bittersweet chocolate, chopped + extra to top
- 1 tablespoon tapioca flour
- 1 egg, at room temperature
- ¼ teaspoon fine sea salt
- Flaky salt to top

- Combine butter and about 4 ounces of chopped chocolate in a heavy saucepan and place the saucepan over low flame
- Cook until chocolate melts. Stir often. The mixture should not be very hot but just warm. Turn off the heat
- Add eggs, salt and sugar into the mixing bowl of the stand mixer. Fit the paddle attachment and set the speed to medium-high and whip until creamy
- Reduce the speed to low and add vanilla. Beat until just incorporated
- Add melted chocolate and beat well Next goes in the flour and beat until well incorporate. Add remaining chopped chocolate fold gently
- Let the batter sit for 10 minutes
- Place mounds of the batter on the prepared baking sheets. You should have 15 cookies in all, so adjust the batter accordingly. Leave sufficient gap between the cookies
- Press a few chocolate pieces on the cookies. Sprinkle flaky salt on the cookies
- Bake the cookies in an oven preheated to 350°F, for about 10 minutes or until firm around the edges
- Let the cookies cool on the baking sheet for 10 minutes. Remove the cookies from the baking sheet and place on a wire rack to cool
- Once completely cooled, place the cookies in an airtight container. It can last for about 3 days

Coffee Ice Cream

Ingredients:

- 1 can (13.6 ounces) coconut milk, chilled
- ¾ cups strong brewed coffee, chilled
- 1 teaspoon vanilla extract
- 1/3 cup maple syrup
- ½ tablespoon instant coffee granules

Instructions:

- Open the can of coconut milk and scoop the coconut cream floating on top
- Add the coconut cream, coffee, instant coffee, maple syrup and vanilla into a blender and blend until smooth
- Pour into a freezer safe container. Cover the container and freeze until semi-frozen. Whisk with an electric hand mixer until creamy
- Freeze until use

Ingredients:

- 5 ounces frozen strawberries, unsweetened, thawed
- 2 tablespoons water
- 1 ½ tablespoons granule stevia-erythritol blend
- 1 teaspoon fresh lemon juice
- ¾ teaspoon unflavoured, powdered gelatine
- ½ cup heavy whipping cream

it. Let it for 5 minutes

- Meanwhile the gelatine is soaked for 5 minutes, add sweetener and place the mixture over medium flame. Stir often, until well combined and dissolves completely
- With the blender machine running on low speed, pour the gelatine mixture through the feeder tube. Blend until well combined
- Pour into a bowl and place the bowl in the refrigerator
- While the mixture is chilling, pour cream into another bowl and whip until soft peaks are formed
- Add one third of the whipped cream into the chilled mixture and fold gently
- Add the rest of the whipped cream and swirl the cream into the mixture for double coloured mousse or mix gently into the mixture until fully incorporated
- Chill until use

2 cups =	1 pint	4 quarts =	1 gallon	3 feet =	1 yard
16 ounces =	1 pint	8 quarts =	2 gallons or 1 peck	5.5 yards =	1 rod
4 cups =	1 quart			40 rods =	1 furlong
1 gill =	1/2 cup or 1/4 pint	4 pecks =	8 gallons or 1 bushel	8 furlongs (5280 feet) =	1 mile
2 pints =	1 quart	16 ounces =	1 pound	6080 feet =	1 nautical mile
4 quarts =	1 gallon	2000 lbs. =	1 ton		
31.5 gal. =	1 barrel				

		Conversion of US Weight and Mass Measure to Metric System		Conversion of US Linear Measure to Metric System	
3 tsp =	1 tbsp			1 inch =	2.54 centimeters
2 tbsp =	1/8 cup or 1 fluid ounce	.0353 ounces =	1 gram		
4 tbsp =	1/4 cup	1/4 ounce =	7 grams	1 foot =	.3048 meters
8 tbsp =	1/2 cup	1 ounce =	28.35 grams	1 yard =	.9144 meters
1 pinch =	1/8 tsp or less	4 ounces =	113.4 grams	1 mile =	1609.3 meters or 1.6093 kilometers
1 tsp =	60 drops	8 ounces =	226.8 grams		
		1 pound =	454 grams	.03937 in. =	1 millimeter

Conversion of US Liquid Measure to Metric System

		2.2046 pounds =	1 kilogram	.3937 in.=	1 centimeter
1 fluid oz. =	29.573 milliliters	.98421 long ton or 1.1023 short tons =	1 metric ton	3.937 in.=	1 decimeter
1 cup =	230 milliliters			39.37 in.=	1 meter
1 quart =	.94635 liters			3280.8 ft. or .62137 miles =	1 kilometer
1 gallon =	3.7854 liters				

.033814 fluid ounce = 1 milliliter

3.3814 fluid ounces = 1 deciliter

33.814 fluid oz. or 1.0567 qt.= 1 liter

To convert a Fahrenheit temperature to Centigrade, do the following:
a. Subtract 32   b. Multiply by 5   c. Divide by 9

To convert Centigrade to Fahrenheit, do the following:
a. Multiply by 9   b. Divide by 5   c. Add 32

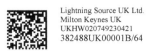
Lightning Source UK Ltd.
Milton Keynes UK
UKHW020749230421
382488UK00001B/64